This journal is intended for personal development and educational purposes only. It is not a substitute for professional mental health care or therapy. If you are experiencing significant emotional distress, please seek help from a licensed mental health professional.

For permissions or inquiries, please contact:
■ [info@familycounselingandcoaching.com
⊕ www.familycounselingandcoaching.com
Printed in the United States of America
First Edition, 2025
ISBN: 979-8-9990778-2-0

Welcome

Welcome to your 30-Day Journey of Empowerment, a practical and transformative tool designed to help you harness the power of your executive functions and navigate daily life with greater focus, consistency, and ease. Whether you're managing ADHD, struggling to maintain habits, or simply seeking to create a more organized and intentional life, this journey is here to support you every step of the way.

This is not about perfection or rigid, one-size-fits-all routines. It's about understanding your unique brain, embracing small, sustainable habits, and building personal systems that align with how you think and operate. You don't have to fight against yourself. Instead, the goal is to work with your mind—recognizing and leveraging its strengths, while gently addressing the challenges you may face.

At the heart of this journey are executive functions—the mental processes that help us manage time, stay organized, regulate impulses, and adapt to changing situations. For many, especially those with ADHD, these functions can be challenging to strengthen. But that doesn't mean they're impossible to improve. In fact, just like any skill, with practice and intention, you can develop and fine-tune these functions to work for you, not against you.

Over the next 30 days, you'll engage with a collection of simple but powerful exercises, prompts, and reflections designed to help you gradually build and strengthen these essential skills. Consistency over perfection is the key phrase here—small steps each day lead to meaningful progress. As you move through this journey, you'll gain the tools to improve focus, follow-through, time management, emotional regulation, and so much more.

This journey is about growth, self-compassion, and empowerment. It's about acknowledging where you are right now, without judgment, and committing to progress, however incremental. The truth is, the path to better self-discipline isn't a straight line, but each small effort compounds into lasting change. And as you improve these skills, you'll find that life becomes more manageable, fulfilling, and aligned with your true potential.

So take a deep breath, turn the page, and let's begin. You're already on the right path.

About the Author

Ernesto Felipe-Cuervo (Ernie Felipe) is a Licensed Mental Health Counselor with advanced degrees in biology (M.S. in Cell Biology) and education (M.S. in Mental Health Counseling). He specializes in emotional regulation, anxiety, trauma, family dynamics, relationship issues, recovery, and anger management. Ernesto is also trained in trauma treatment, Rapid Resolution Therapy, and Acceptance and Commitment Therapy (ACT). In addition to his private practice, Ernesto coaches individuals of all ages, helping them transform life's challenges into opportunities for growth through self-compassion and values-based action. His coaching approach is also informed by training in the development of executive functioning skills, including time management, organization, and goal-directed behavior. Before working full-time in private practice, he spent over 12 years as Director of School Counseling at a private school in Miami, where he supported students, parents, and teachers through emotional and educational challenges. Ernesto has also led workshops on communication, parenting, and family dynamics for churches, local and international organizations.

Table of Contents

Welcome...Page 2

About the Author..Page 3

Introduction to Executive Skills ....Page 5

Self-Awareness ....Page 8

Time Awareness ....Page 10

The Starting Line ....Page 12

Finish What You Started ....Page 14

Accept the Discomfort ....Page 16

Urges vs. Actions ....Page 18

Weekly Check-In ....Page 20

Gaining Momentum ....Page 22

The Planning Mind ....Page 24

No Mess, Less Stress ....Page 26

Strength in Flexibility ....Page 28

What Matters Most ....Page 30

Focus Anchors ....Page 32

Weekly Check-In ....Page 34

To Do or Not to Do ....Page 36

Speaking Up for Yourself ....Page 38

From Dreaming to Doing ....Page 40

Emotional Energy ....Page 42

One Task, One Focus ....Page 44

The Power of Pause ....Page 46

Weekly Check-In ....Page 48

The When Plan ....Page 50

Self-Compassion Check ....Page 52

Triggers and Transitions ....Page 54

Reward Your Brain ....Page 56

Brain Dumps and Lists ....Page 58

Default to Done ....Page 60

Emotional Forecasting ....Page 62

Celebrate Effort ....Page 64

The Purpose Identity ....Page 66

Appendix: Executive Skills Questionnaire ....Page 68

Final Words..Page 76

🛠 What Are Executive Skills?

There are several core executive function skills, and each one plays a unique role in how we plan, start, and complete tasks. These include response inhibition, working memory, emotional regulation, sustained attention, task initiation, planning and prioritization, organization, time management, goal-directed persistence, flexibility, and metacognition. Think of them as a toolkit: some tools might be sharp and reliable, while others are rusty or harder to access when you need them. Everyone's profile is different — and that's perfectly okay. Each person has unique strengths and areas where they may struggle more, and that variation is part of what makes us human. The goal isn't to master all of these skills overnight or to compare yourself to others. Instead, it's about becoming more aware of where you excel and where you might need support, so you can make intentional, positive changes. This journey is about growth, not perfection, and each step forward brings you closer to becoming a more empowered version of yourself—one that works with your natural abilities and challenges to thrive.

🔍 Key Skills That Affect Daily Discipline

Let's break down a few of these skills. Response inhibition helps you pause before acting — essential for resisting distractions or impulsive decisions. Working memory allows you to hold information in your mind while using it, like remembering steps in a task. Emotional regulation helps you manage frustration or overwhelm without shutting down. If these are areas of struggle, self-discipline can feel harder — not because you're lazy, but because the brain systems that support restraint and calm under pressure need more intentional support.

📌 Focus, Start, and Follow Through

Sustained attention allows you to stay focused over time, especially on tasks that aren't naturally interesting. Task initiation is the skill that helps you start something without endless delay — even when it's hard. Planning and prioritization involve setting goals and deciding what matters most, especially when time or energy are limited. Without these, it's easy to feel scattered or overwhelmed by competing responsibilities. But these skills can be developed with practice — especially when approached in small, manageable steps.

▮ Staying Organized & On Track

Organization and time management help you stay on top of tasks, items, and commitments. Struggles here can lead to missed deadlines or underestimating how long things take. But with routines, visual cues, and structured support, the mental load gets lighter. The key is to work with your brain—not against it. Small adjustments can create lasting change.

● Persistence and Progress

Goal-directed persistence helps you keep going, even when things are hard or the rewards aren't immediate. It's key for self-discipline, especially during low-motivation moments. Some thrive on internal drive; others need external support—both are valid. What matters is knowing what helps you stay consistent. This journal will guide you in discovering and strengthening that support system over time.

▮ Adapt and Reflect

Flexibility and metacognition complete the toolkit. Flexibility lets you adapt when plans change, boosting resilience. Metacognition helps you reflect on your thinking—asking what works and what doesn't. These advanced skills grow with intentional reflection and self-awareness, which this journal is designed to nurture. Developing them can lead to greater control and calm in daily life.

♟ Your Brain, Your Blueprint

Everyone's executive function profile is unique. Some people excel at planning and setting goals but struggle with managing their emotions. Others may find it easy to get started on tasks but have difficulty staying organized or managing their time effectively. This doesn't mean you're incapable or failing—it simply means your path to self-discipline and success needs to be tailored to your individual brain. The more you learn about how your mind works, the better you can develop strategies that truly support you. Embracing both your strengths and challenges is essential for meaningful growth and lasting progress.

✎ How This Journal Helps

Throughout this journal,

- You will reflect on your habits, track your progress, and explore what helps you stay focused and committed.
- You will be encouraged to notice small victories, celebrate effort, and build sustainable habits instead of chasing perfect results.
- You will learn to develop curiosity about your innate abilities, work with your strengths, and gently support your challenges—not ignore them or judge them.

This journal may not be for everyone. It might not be for you—although this system is often incredibly helpful for those who are tired of being labeled lazy or distracted.
It is especially valuable for people who have begun to recognize their own unique talents and strengths—gifts only they possess—that can lead them toward the life they want.
Everything changes when you become aware of those inner resources and learn to use them more effectively, in ways that align with what truly drives you.

🚀 Moving Forward

This isn't the end — it's just the beginning. Self-discipline isn't about control; it's about returning to what matters and creating an environment where you can follow through. That means experimenting, being kind to yourself, and recognizing that progress is rarely linear. You're building a foundation that supports your goals, your values, and your well-being. This journal will walk with you — one intentional, doable step at a time.

To support your work in this journal, we've included a questionnaire at the end based on common behaviors that help or hinder self-discipline across executive skills. It's not a diagnostic tool, but a guide to help you focus your efforts over the next 30 days.

Have a rewarding journey of discovery and growth. 🌱

Day 1   *Self Awareness*

🗨 **Focus Skill: Metacognition**

"Knowing yourself is the beginning of all wisdom." – Aristotle

🧍⬛ **Target Behavior Identification**

Which self-awareness challenges show up most for you?

_____

_____

_____

Suggested Target Behaviors:

- Notice a habit in the moment (e.g., biting nails, zoning out, avoiding)
- Identify what triggers your procrastination or distraction
- Pause and ask yourself, "What am I doing and why?"
- Observe your mood or energy changes throughout the day

My Target Behavior for Today

_____

⬛ **Suggested Activity (3 Steps)**

- Pause mid-task and ask: "What am I feeling? What am I doing?"
- Write down one unhelpful habit or thought you noticed today.
- Write a more helpful replacement thought or response.

■ Evaluation System

Rate yourself based on insight gained:

● Green (Clear Insight): I noticed a pattern and wrote it down.
● Yellow (Some Insight): I paused but struggled to name the behavior.
● Red (No Insight): I didn't stop to reflect today.

Reflection:

What surprised me about my behavior today? What helped me stay focused? What can I do differently tomorrow?

_____

_____

_____

_____

_____

_____

Day 2 — *Time Awaereness*

🗨 **Focus Skill: Time management**

"Time is what we want most, but what we use worst." – William Penn

👤⬛ **Target Behavior Identification**

Which time distortion behaviors apply to you?

_____

_____

_____

Suggested Target Behaviors:

- Estimate time needed for one common task today (like email, getting ready)
- Notice how often you check the clock or forget to
- Set reminders before a transition and see how well they help
- Write down how long you think a task will take—then compare

My Target Behavior for Today

_____

⬛ **Suggested Activity (3 Steps)**

- Choose one task and estimate how long it will take.
- Set a timer and track the actual time.
- Compare your estimate to reality and write the difference.

■ Evaluation System

Rate yourself based on insight gained:

● Green (Clear Insight): I noticed a pattern and wrote it down.
● Yellow (Some Insight): I paused but struggled to name the behavior.
● Red (No Insight): I didn't stop to reflect today.

Reflection:

What surprised me about my behavior today? What helped me stay focused? What can I do differently tomorrow? What threw off my time estimation? What distracted me the most? What small win am I proud of today?

_____

_____

_____

_____

_____

_____

Day 3

The Starting Line

▌ Focus Skill: Task Initiation

"You don't have to be great to start, but you have to start to be great."
– Zig Ziglar

▮▌ Target Behavior Identification

Pick one habit that blocks you from getting started.

_____

_____

_____

Suggested Target Behaviors:

- Avoiding a task because it feels too big or unclear
- Overthinking the first step
- Waiting for the "right" time or perfect conditions
- Getting stuck in preparation instead of action

My Target Behavior for Today

_____

▌ Suggested Activity (3 Steps)

- Choose one task you've been avoiding (email, workout, writing, etc.).
- Break it down to the smallest possible first step (e.g., open document, put on shoes).
- Do just the first step and count that as a win — bonus if you keep going.

12

■ Evaluation System

Rate yourself based on insight gained:

● Green (Clear Action): I identified a task I've been avoiding, broke it down, and completed the first step — bonus if I kept going.
● Yellow (Partial Follow-Through): I thought about the task and the first step, but didn't take action
● Red (No Action): I avoided the task and didn't attempt to break it down.

Reflection:

"Today, I took the first step toward _____. What helped me begin was _____. Next time, I'll remember that _____."

_____

_____

_____

_____

_____

_____

Day 4

Finishing What You Started

▌ Focus Skill: Task Completion

"It always seems impossible until it's done." – Nelson Mandela

♦ ▌ Target Behavior Identification

Pick one habit that blocks you from completing tasks.

_____

_____

_____

Suggested Target Behaviors:

- Leaving tasks half-finished once they lose momentum
- Getting distracted by new ideas or responsibilities
- Striving for perfection and never feeling "done"
- Avoiding the final step because of fear of judgment or outcome

My Target Behavior for Today

_____

▌ Suggested Activity (3 Steps)

- Choose one small task you've started but haven't finished.
- Set a timer for 10–15 minutes and focus only on completing what's left.
- When the timer ends, check it off—done is better than perfect.

14

■ Evaluation System

Rate yourself based on insight gained:

● Green: Chose an unfinished task, set a timer, focused, and finished it.
● Yellow: Chose a task but didn't finish or got distracted
● Red: Didn't choose or work on any unfinished task.

Reflection:

Today I finished _____, and what helped me complete it was _____. Next time I feel stuck, I'll remind myself _____."

_____

_____

_____

_____

_____

_____

Day 5

Accept The Discomfort

♨ Focus Skill: Emotional Regulation

"Discomfort is the price of admission to a meaningful life." – Susan David

🧍⬛ Target Behavior Identification

What discomfort do you usually avoid?

_____

_____

_____

Suggested Target Behaviors:

- Stay with a boring task for at least 5 minutes
- Engage in a tough conversation instead of avoiding it
- Sit with an overwhelming feeling without numbing (e.g., not checking your phone)
- Identify the emotion that's driving procrastination today

My Target Behavior for Today

_____

⬛ Suggested Activity (3 Steps)

- When discomfort shows up, name the emotion (e.g., "I feel frustrated").
- Set a 5-minute timer and stay with the task.
- Journal briefly about what you noticed (without judgment).

■ Evaluation System

Rate yourself based on insight gained:

● Green (Stayed With It): I noticed discomfort and stayed.
● Yellow (Halfway): I started but needed a break.
● Red (Avoided): I escaped the task or numbed out.

Reflection:

"When I felt _____, I chose to stay. What I noticed during those 5 minutes was _____. Next time, I want to remember _____."

_____

_____

_____

_____

_____

_____

Day 6

Urges vs. Actions

⚖️ Focus Skill: Impulse Control

"Between stimulus and response, there is a space... and in that space is our power to choose." – Viktor Frankl

🧍⬛ Target Behavior Identification

What impulse do you want to manage better?

_____

_____

_____

Suggested Target Behaviors:

- Pause before checking your phone
- Avoid blurting out in conversations
- Resist online shopping or impulse decisions
- Delay a snack or craving to test your response
- Wait 5 seconds before reacting to a trigger

My Target Behavior for Today

_____

⬛ Suggested Activity (3 Steps)

- Pause and Notice the Urge (Before reacting, take a moment to identify the impulse, or say to yourself: "I want to _____."
- Engage in a Mindful Practice by using 5-4-3-2-1 sensory grounding, boxed breathing (inhale-hold-exhale-hold, for 7-4-11 seconds each, brief meditation or body scan)
- Choose a Different Response (don't act on the urge, try a new, intentional response).

◼ Evaluation System

Rate yourself based on insight gained:

● Green (Redirected the Impulse): I paused and made a better choice.
● Yellow (Partially Aware): I noticed too late but reflected.
● Red (Automatic Response): I acted without awareness.

Reflection:

What did you notice when you paused, named the urge, and chose a different response instead of reacting automatically?

_____

_____

_____

_____

_____

_____

Day 7

Weekly Check-In

■ **Focus Skill: Self-Monitoring**

"Success is the sum of small efforts, repeated day in and day out."
– Robert Collier

👤■ **Target Behavior Identification**

What habit or area needs more self-tracking?

_____

_____

Suggested Target Behaviors:

- Look for patterns in your mood, motivation, or focus
- Track how often you follow through on a small habit
- Pay attention to language (e.g., "I never get it right")
- Notice your tendency to only see negatives

My Target Behavior for Today

_____

■ **Suggested Activity (3 Steps)**

- Review your journal entries from Days 1–6.
- Write down 1 thing you learned and 1 small win.
- Set one intention for the next 7 days.

■ Evaluation System

Rate yourself based on insight gained:

- ● Green (Clear Insight + Plan): I identified wins and set a goal.
- ● Yellow (Partial): I skimmed but didn't dig deep.
- ● Red (Skipped It): I didn't review or reflect.

Reflection:

What's one theme I noticed this week?

_____

_____

_____

_____

_____

_____

Day 8
Gaining Momentum

🏆 **Focus Skill: Motivation**

"The journey of a thousand miles begins with one step." – Lao Tzu

🚹⬛ **Target Behavior Identification**

What prevents you from recognizing progress?

_____

_____

_____

Suggested Target Behaviors:

- Track completion of one small task today
- Acknowledge even minor effort (e.g., starting, trying again)
- Avoid comparing yourself to others
- Practice saying "That was enough for today"

My Target Behavior for Today

_____

⬛ **Suggested Activity (3 Steps)**

- List 3 small wins from this week (effort counts!).
- Pick one and describe why it matters.
- Reward yourself (e.g., a break, music, a high-five).

■ Evaluation System

Rate yourself based on insight gained:

● Green (Named & Celebrated): I felt good about my wins.
● Yellow (Wrote but Minimized): I listed them but didn't feel them.
● Red (Skipped It): I couldn't name any wins.

Reflection:

How did it feel to focus on effort instead of outcome? What part of the process felt most engaging? What did I enjoy or notice while doing the work, not just finishing it?

_____

_____

_____

_____

_____

_____

Day 9

The Planning Mind

📖 Focus Skill: Planning

"A goal without a plan is just a wish." – Antoine de Saint-Exupéry

🧍⬛ Target Behavior Identification

What's your biggest challenge with planning?

_____

_____

_____

Suggested Target Behaviors:

- Avoid feeling overwhelmed by large tasks by breaking them down into small steps.
- Break the habit of getting stuck without taking action by using the "If-Then" planning (for example, "If I feel stuck, then ___").
- Stop planning the entire project at once, focusing only on the next step.

My Target Behavior for Today

_____

⬛ Suggested Activity (3 Steps)

- Pick one avoided task.
- Break it into 3 tiny steps (under 10 minutes each).
- Schedule one step for today.

◼ Evaluation System

Rate yourself based on insight gained:

● Green (Planned + Did It): I made and followed a micro-plan.
● Yellow (Planned but Didn't Act): I planned but avoided the task.
● Red (Didn't Plan): I skipped breaking it down.

Reflection:

hat helped or blocked me from following my plan? How did I adjust when things didn't go as expected? What can I do differently tomorrow to stay aligned with my goals?

_____

_____

_____

_____

_____

Day 10

No Mess Less Stress

⚒ Focus Skill: Organization

"You can't reach for anything new if your hands are still full of yesterday's clutter." – Louise Smith

🧍⬛ Target Behavior Identification

Which area of your environment could use some help?

_____

_____

Suggested Target Behaviors:

- Clear visual clutter from your workspace
- Organize one digital folder or your browser tabs
- Add a visual anchor like a checklist or sticky note
- Prep tomorrow's essentials in advance (e.g., keys, clothes)

My Target Behavior for Today

_____

⬛ Suggested Activity (3 Steps)

- Pick one small space (desk corner, bag, desktop) to reset.
- Remove 3 things that don't belong.
- Add 1 visual cue that supports focus (post-it, checklist, timer).

26

■ Evaluation System

Rate yourself based on insight gained:

● Green (Cleared + Added Cues): I made a change and felt the shift.
● Yellow (Cleared Only): I tidied but didn't add focus tools.
● Red (No Change): I didn't adjust my space.

Reflection:

What environment helps me focus best? What distractions tend to pull me away? What changes can I make to create a more focus-friendly space tomorrow?

_____

_____

_____

_____

_____

_____

DATE: / /

Day 11

Strength in Flexibility

⟆ Focus Skill: Cognitive Flexibility

"The reed that bends in the wind is stronger than the oak that breaks in a storm." — Chinese Proverb

🛈 Target Behavior Identification
What makes change or unpredictability hard?

_____

_____

_____

Suggested Target Behaviors:

- Adapt calmly when plans change.
- Transition between tasks with greater ease and openness.
- Adjust routines smoothly when needed.

My Target Behavior for Today

_____

◼ Suggested Activity (3 Steps)

- Think of one thing today that might not go as planned.
- Choose a backup plan or flexible response in advance.
- If a change happens, pause and try the new plan.

■ Evaluation System

Rate yourself based on insight gained:

- ● Green (Adapted with Ease): I adjusted and kept going.
- ● Yellow (Struggled but Tried): I resisted but attempted flexibility.
- ● Red (Shut Down): I felt stuck and didn't adjust.

Reflexion:

What helped or hurt my ability to pivot? What "color" best describes how I adapted today? What could help me move toward green next time?

_____

_____

_____

_____

_____

_____

Day 12

What Matters Most

● **Focus Skill: Prioritizing**

"The key is not to prioritize what's on your schedule, but to schedule your priorities." – Stephen R. Covey

🧍■ **Target Behavior Identification**
What gets in the way of knowing what to do first?

_____

_____

_____

Suggested Target Behaviors:

- I treat everything like it's urgent.
- I avoid harder tasks even when they're more important.
- I jump between tasks based on mood, not impact.
- I say "yes" to everything, even when my plate is full.
- I underestimate how long tasks will take and overcommit myself.

My Target Behavior for Today

_____

■ **Suggested Activity (3 Steps)**

- Write down 3 things you feel you should do today.
- Circle the one that would have the biggest impact if done.
- Do that one thing first—or block time on your calendar for it.

◼ Evaluation System

Did I identify and focus on my true priority?

- ● Green (Focused): I chose a top priority and acted on it.
- ● Yellow (Planned but Scattered): I picked a priority but didn't follow through.
- ● Red (Unfocused): I didn't pick or act on a clear priority.

Reflection:

What helped (or hurt) my ability to focus on what matters today? What did I choose to give my time to — and did it align with what I truly value?

_____

_____

_____

_____

_____

_____

Day 13

Focus Anchors

● Focus Skill: Sustained Attention

"Where your attention goes, your energy flows." – Tony Robbins

♦ ■ Target Behavior Identification

What tends to distract me most?

_____

_____

_____

Suggested Target Behaviors:

- I switch tasks constantly.
- I work in a distracting environment.
- I forget what I was doing mid-task.
- I start my day without a clear plan.
- I try to multitask instead of focusing on one thing at a time.

My Target Behavior for Today

_____

■ Suggested Activity (3 Steps)

- Choose one task you want to stay focused on.
- Use a "focus anchor" like a timer, music, or checklist.
- When distracted, gently return to the task using your anchor.

■ Evaluation System
Was I able to sustain attention?

- Green (Stayed With It): I used an anchor and stayed focused.
- Yellow (Distracted But Returned): I got off track but redirected.
- Red (Constantly Distracted): I couldn't stay with the task.

Reflection:

What anchor helped me the most? When did I notice it keeping me grounded? How can I make it more accessible next time?

_____

_____

_____

_____

_____

Day 14

Weekly Check-In

■ **Focus Skill: Self-Reflection**

"Study the past if you would define the future." — Confucius

🚶■ **Target Behavior Identification**

What reflection habits do I need to build?

_____

_____

_____

Suggested Target Behaviors:

- I skip self-reflection and repeat patterns.
- I judge myself instead of being curious.
- I forget what worked in previous days.
- I rush ahead without pausing to learn from setbacks.
- I focus on what I didn't do, instead of what I did accomplish.

My Target Behavior for Today

_____

■ **Suggested Activity (3 Steps)**

- Review Days 8–13 and circle what worked.
- Identify one area that still needs work.
- Write one kind and curious question to explore next week.

■ Evaluation System
Did I reflect effectively?

● Green (Planned + Did It): I made and followed a micro-plan.
● Yellow (Planned but Didn't Act): I planned but avoided the task.
● Red (Didn't Plan): I skipped breaking it down.

Reflection:

How can I approach next week with more intention? What small shift would make the biggest difference? Where did I feel most aligned — or misaligned — with my values this week, and how can that guide my next steps?

_____

_____

_____

_____

_____

_____

Day 15

To do or not to do?

● **Focus Skill: Decision Making**

"The risk of a wrong decision is preferable to the terror of indecision."
– Maimonides

👤■ **Target Behavior Identification**
What makes decision-making difficult for me?

_____

_____

_____

Suggested Target Behaviors:

- I get stuck overthinking options.
- I fear making the wrong choice.
- I avoid decisions because I'm unsure of the outcome.
- I delay action waiting for the "perfect" option.
- I second-guess choices I've already made.

My Target Behavior for Today

_____

■ **Suggested Activity (3 Steps)**

- Identify one decision you've been putting off (big or small).
- Write down 2-3 pros and cons of each option.
- Choose one option and commit to it, even if you're uncertain.

■ Evaluation System

Did I make a decision today?

● Green (Decided): I made a choice and stuck with it.
● Yellow (Hesitant): I made a decision but felt uncertain.
● Red (Indecisive): I couldn't make a decision today.

Reflection:

How did making a decision affect my anxiety or stress levels? What did I notice in my body or thoughts before, during, and after choosing? Did the act of deciding bring relief, regret, clarity — or something else?

_____

_____

_____

_____

_____

_____

Day 16

Speaking Up for Yourself

♟ Focus Skill: Self-Advocacy

"Our lives begin to end the day we become silent about things that matter."
— Martin Luther King Jr.

♦ ■ Target Behavior Identification

"Why is it so hard for me to speak up for myself?"

_____

_____

_____

Suggested Target Behaviors:

- I feel uncomfortable asking for help.
- I fear being judged or misunderstood.
- I worry about appearing weak or incapable.
- I assume others are too busy to support me.
- I downplay my needs to avoid feeling like a burden.

My Target Behavior for Today

_____

■ Suggested Activity (3 Steps)

- Identify a situation where you need support or clarity and plan how you will express your need (clearly and confidently).
- Rehearse in front of the mirror no less than 5 times
- Speak up and ask for what you need and role-play answering yourself back.

■ Evaluation System

Did I speak up for myself today?

● Green (Advocated): I spoke up and got the support I needed.
● Yellow (Planned but Hesitated): I planned but didn't fully advocate for myself.
● Red (Silent): I didn't speak up at all.

Reflection:

"How did speaking up for myself affect my confidence or stress? What made it easier to speak up—and what held me back?"

_____

_____

_____

_____

_____

_____

Day 17
From Dreaming to Doing

⬤ Focus Skill: Goal Setting

"The best way to predict your future is to create it." – Abraham Lincoln

🧍⬛ Target Behavior Identification

"Why is it hard for me to make a plan and stick to it?"

_____

_____

_____

Suggested Target Behaviors:

- I'm not sure what my goals should be.
- It it easier to dream than to actually start?
- Something stops me from breaking big dreams into small steps?
- I feel overwhelmed by long-term goals.
- I avoid setting goals because I'm afraid I won't achieve them.

My Target Behavior for Today

_____

⬛ Suggested Activity (3 Steps)

- Write down 3 things that truly matter to you (e.g., education, personal growth, stability).
- Pick one value and turn it into a small, specific action you can do this week (e.g., education → register for school or research enrollment deadlines).
- After doing it, reflect on what happened and how it felt (e.g., "I felt relieved and more in control after taking the first step").

■ Evaluation System

Did I take action toward my goals today?

● Green (Action Taken): I made progress by completing a specific step toward my goal (e.g., registered for school or took the first step in researching).
● Yellow (Planned but Hesitated): I planned to take action but didn't fully follow through (e.g., I thought about registering but didn't).
● Red (No Action): I didn't take any steps toward my goal today (e.g., I didn't research or register at all).

Reflection:

What influenced my ability to take action today? Was I held back by lack of time, unclear steps, or feeling overwhelmed? What obstacles or wins stood out — and how can that insight help me move forward tomorrow?

_____

_____

_____

_____

_____

Day 18

Emotional Energy

● Focus Skill: Goal Setting

"Name it to tame it." – Dr. Dan Siegel

♦■ Target Behavior Identification

What emotions interfere with focus and discipline?

_____

_____

Suggested Target Behaviors:

- I avoid tasks that bring up anxiety or frustration.
- I push through emotions without naming them.
- I overreact to small stressors.
- I shut down or procrastinate when I feel overwhelmed.
- I seek quick comfort (e.g., scrolling, snacking) instead of facing discomfort.

My Target Behavior for Today

_____

■ Suggested Activity (3 Steps)

- Pause and identify one emotion you felt today.
- Name it using the sentence: "I feel ___ because ___."
- Choose a healthy action (deep breath, stretch, journaling, ask for help).

■ Evaluation System
How well did I manage my emotional energy?

- ● Green (Named + Navigated): I identified and responded with care.
- ● Yellow (Felt It, Then Reacted): I noticed but didn't redirect.
- ● Red (Overwhelmed): I let the emotion control the moment.

Reflection:

What emotions tend to derail my focus the most (e.g., anxiety, boredom, frustration)? What's my usual response when I feel those emotions during a task? What helped me stay grounded or refocus when I got emotional?

_____

_____

_____

_____

_____

_____

Day 19

One Task, One Focus

🎧 Focus Skill: Attention Control

"The successful warrior is the average man, with laser-like focus." – Bruce Lee

🧍⬛ Target Behavior Identification

What habits make it hard to focus on one thing?

_____

_____

_____

Suggested Target Behaviors:

- I multitask constantly.
- I switch tabs or apps without finishing.
- I rarely complete something before starting another.
- I get distracted easily and forget what I was originally doing.
- I start tasks impulsively without planning or prioritizing.

My Target Behavior for Today

_____

⬛ Suggested Activity (3 Steps)

- Pick one task to complete without switching.
- Close or remove all distractions (tabs, devices, alerts).
- Set a short timer (10–15 mins) and commit to staying on task until it ends.

◼ Evaluation System

Did I stay with one task?

- ● Green (Stayed the Whole Time): I resisted switching and stayed focused.
- ● Yellow (Switched Briefly): I switched but came back.
- ● Red (Task Hopping): I couldn't stay with one task.

Reflection:

What helped or hurt my ability to stay focused? What was happening around me when I lost focus? What thoughts or emotions pulled my attention away from the task?

_____

_____

_____

_____

_____

Day 20

The Power of Pause

■ Focus Skill: Impulse Control

"Like a city whose walls are broken through is a person who lacks self-control."
— Proverbs 25:28

♦■ Target Behavior Identification

What impulsive reactions show up most for me?

_____

_____

_____

Suggested Target Behaviors:

- I interrupt conversations.
- I click or scroll when uncomfortable.
- I make snap decisions I regret.
- I avoid difficult conversations or topics.
- I react impulsively instead of taking time to consider my response.

My Target Behavior for Today

_____

■ Suggested Activity (3 Steps)

- Choose one moment where you're likely to react impulsively.
- Practice a "pause phrase" like: "Stop, Pause-Decide" or "Breath-Evaluate-Act."
- Decide your next step after the pause—not during the urge.

■ Evaluation System

How did I handle impulse moments?

● Green (Paused + Chose): I paused and responded thoughtfully.
● Yellow (Caught It Late): I noticed but paused after the fact.
● Red (Acted on Urge): I didn't pause or redirect.

Reflection:

What emotion appeared when I felt the urge to react? How did my behavior change when I used a pause phrase? What did I learn about myself by waiting before acting?

_____

_____

_____

_____

_____

Day 21

Weekly Check-In

● **Focus Skill: Reflection**

"Reflection turns experience into wisdom." – John C. Maxwell

👤■ **Target Behavior Identification**

Where have I notice I tend to resist reflection?

_____

_____

_____

Suggested Target Behaviors:

- I skip check-ins because they feel unimportant.
- I only notice what went wrong.
- I reflect but don't make adjustments.
- I judge my progress instead of learning from it.
- I rush past wins without acknowledging them.

My Target Behavior for Today

_____

■ **Suggested Activity (3 Steps)**

- Write 3 things that went well this week.
- Identify 1 thing that felt difficult or frustrating.
- Write 1 change or strategy to try next week.

■ Evaluation System

Did I complete my reflection?

- Green (Full Check-In): I reflected and wrote all 3 parts.
- Yellow (Partial Effort): I reflected but skipped something.
- Red (Skipped It): I didn't do a check-in today.

Reflection:

What did this reflection reveal that I hadn't noticed? How might this new awareness influence my actions moving forward? What steps can I take to stay mindful of this insight?

_____

_____

_____

_____

_____

_____

Day 22

The When Plan

📋 Focus Skill: Time Management

"If it's not scheduled, it's not real." – Marie Forleo

🧍⬛ Target Behavior Identification

What stops me from planning effectively?

_____

_____

_____

Suggested Target Behaviors:

- I don't assign times to tasks.
- I wing it and forget things.
- I avoid planning because it feels rigid.
- I underestimate how long things will take and fall behind.
- I jump into tasks without a clear order or priority.

My Target Behavior for Today

_____

⬛ Suggested Activity (3 Steps)

- Pick two important tasks: one ongoing and one for today or tomorrow.
- Choose a specific time or times during the week to do one and complete the other (not just "sometime").
- Put it in your calendar, planner, or phone alert.

■ Evaluation System

Did I follow through with my time plan?

- ● Green (Planned + Did It): I scheduled and followed through.
- ● Yellow (Scheduled, Shifted): I planned but changed the time.
- ● Red (Didn't Do It): I didn't schedule or follow through

Reflection:

How did scheduling the when change my sense of control? What felt easier once I gave my task a time? What resistance came up when I tried to plan ahead?

_____

_____

_____

_____

_____

_____

Day 23

Self-Compassion Check

♥ **Focus Skill: Emotional Regulation**

"Procrastination is not laziness; it's fear. Call it by its name and forgive yourself." — Julia Cameron

🧍⬛ **Target Behavior Identification**

How do I treat myself when I fall short?

_____

_____

_____

Suggested Target Behaviors:

- I call myself lazy or bad.
- I shut down or spiral.
- I push harder without rest or grace.
- I ignore my limits until I burn out.
- I compare myself to others and feel like I'm always behind.

My Target Behavior for Today

_____

⬛ **Suggested Activity (3 Steps)**

- Catch a moment you felt overwhelmed or off track.
- Practice saying to yourself: "It's okay not to have everything figured out."
- Do one kind thing for yourself (pause, reset, or ask for help)

■ Evaluation System

Did I show myself compassion?

- ● Green (Responded with Kindness): I talked to myself gently and adjusted.
- ● Yellow (Some Effort): I tried but slipped into harshness.
- ● Red (Self-Blame): I judged myself harshly and didn't redirect.

Reflection:

What changes when I support myself instead of criticize? What does my inner voice sound like when it's kind? How do I act differently when I believe I'm worthy of patience?

_____

_____

_____

_____

_____

_____

Day 24

Triggers and Transitions

■ **Focus Skill: Flexibility**

"Life is 10% what happens to us and 90% how we react." – Charles Swindoll

👤■ **Target Behavior Identification**

What transitions or triggers knock me off track?

_____

_____

Suggested Target Behaviors:

- I resist switching tasks.
- I get stuck after interruptions.
- I don't handle surprises well.
- I lose momentum when plans change.
- I need extra time to restart after being thrown off.

My Target Behavior for Today

_____

■ **Suggested Activity (3 Steps)**

- Pick one daily transition that's usually hard (like starting homework or ending screen time).
- Choose a simple cue to signal the shift (like standing up, deep breath, or saying "Time to reset").
- Use your cue in the moment and notice how it affects your focus or mood.

■ Evaluation System
Did I handle transitions with more awareness?

- ● Green (Used the Cue + Shifted Well): I transitioned smoothly.
- ● Yellow (Used It, Still Struggled): I tried but it was rough.
- ● Red (No Cue or Shift): I resisted or got stuck.

Reflection:

How does prepping for transitions affect my mood or momentum? What happens when I skip a transition routine? Which transitions feel smoother, and why?

_____

_____

_____

_____

_____

_____

Day 25

Reward Your Brain

🐾 Focus Skill: Motivation
"What is rewarded is repeated." – B.F. Skinner

🚹⬛ Target Behavior Identification
Where do I hold back from giving myself credit or encouragement?

_____

_____

_____

Suggested Target Behaviors:

- I wait for big wins to celebrate.
- I don't reward effort—just outcomes.
- I forget to build in fun or pleasure.
- I downplay my progress even when I'm improving.
- I move to the next task without acknowledging what I just did.

My Target Behavior for Today

_____

⬛ Suggested Activity (3 Steps)

- Identify one meaningful task or habit you want to complete today.
- Choose a simple, healthy reward that genuinely motivates you (like a favorite podcast, a short break, or a treat).
- Follow through by giving yourself the reward right after completing the task—no delays or guilt.

■ Evaluation System

Did I pair reward with effort?

● Green (Did Task + Rewarded): Task complete + reward earned.
● Yellow (Did Task, Forgot Reward): No reward but task done.
● Red (Skipped Task or Reward): I didn't follow through.

Reflection:

What types of rewards truly boost my energy? When do I feel most satisfied after completing something? How can I build in small rewards without feeling guilty or indulgent?

_____

_____

_____

_____

_____

Day 26

Brain Dumps and Lists

🗨 Focus Skill: Working Memory

"Your brain is for having ideas, not holding them." – David Allen

👤⬛ Target Behavior Identification

What do I do instead of externalizing my thoughts?

_____

_____

_____

Suggested Target Behaviors:

- I try to hold everything in my head.
- I forget tasks constantly.
- I write lists but never look at them.
- I feel overwhelmed by trying to remember everything.
- I delay tasks because I can't keep track of everything.

My Target Behavior for Today

_____

⬛ Suggested Activity (3 Steps)

- Set a 5-minute timer. Dump everything on your mind (tasks, worries, reminders) into a notebook or app.
- Pick 3 items that feel most important.
- Create a basic plan or list to address those 3.

■ Evaluation System

Did I offload my mental clutter?

● Green (Dump + Prioritized): I brain dumped and planned.
● Yellow (Dumped but Didn't Use It): I wrote things down but didn't act.
● Red (Didn't Offload): I kept everything in my head.

Reflection:

What changed when I wrote it all down? How did I feel after clearing things from my mind? What did I do differently with a clear plan?

_____

_____

_____

_____

_____

Day 27

Default to Done

◼ Focus Skill: Task Completion

"Done is better than perfect." – Sheryl Sandberg

ⓘ ◼ Target Behavior Identification

What perfectionist habits delay my finish line?

_____

_____

_____

Suggested Target Behaviors:

- I tinker endlessly instead of finishing.
- I avoid turning in or sharing work.
- I wait until something feels "perfect."
- I procrastinate when I feel unsure or overwhelmed.
- I redo things unnecessarily, even when they're already good enough.

My Target Behavior for Today

_____

◼ Suggested Activity (3 Steps)

- Choose one task you've been over-editing, over-thinking, or avoiding.
- Decide what "done enough" looks like (set a clear finish line).
- Complete it and call it done—even if it's imperfect.

■ Evaluation System

Did I finish something instead of perfecting?

● Green (Finished + Let Go): I completed and accepted the result.
● Yellow (Finished, Still Tinkered): I did it but kept tweaking.
● Red (Didn't Finish): I kept postponing or perfecting.

Reflection:

How does "done" feel compared to "perfect"? What am I afraid might happen if I share something that feels unfinished? What would it mean to trust that "good enough" is enough?

_____

_____

_____

_____

_____

_____

Day 28
Emotional Forecasting

☁ Focus Skill: Self-Awareness

"The time to repair the roof is when the sun is shining." – John F. Kennedy

👤⬛ Target Behavior Identification

When, where, and how do my emotions catch me by surprise?

_____

_____

_____

Suggested Target Behaviors:

- I ignore warning signs of stress or fatigue.
- I assume I'll be fine, then I crash.
- I don't plan for emotional triggers.
- I dismiss my need for rest until it's too late.
- I push through discomfort instead of addressing the cause.

My Target Behavior for Today

_____

⬛ Suggested Activity (3 Steps)

- Identify one situation today that may feel emotionally tricky (conflict, overload, low energy).
- Write how you expect to feel and how you want to respond.
- Prepare a backup plan (e.g., take a break, journal, walk away).

■ Evaluation System

Did I anticipate and manage emotions effectively?

- Green (Predicted + Used a Strategy): I forecasted and responded intentionally.
- Yellow (Partially Aware): I noticed but didn't manage well.
- Red (Blindsided): I didn't prepare or reflect at all.

.

Reflection:

What emotions am I likely to encounter that I can learn to make space for, rather than avoid?
How can I respond to these emotions in a way that supports the kind of person I want to be?
What values can guide me when difficult feelings show up?

_____

_____

_____

_____

_____

Day 29

Celebrate Effort

🎉 Focus Skill: Growth Mindset

"You do not rise to the level of your goals. You fall to the level of your systems."
-James Clear

🧍⬛ Target Behavior Identification

Where do I fail to acknowledge my effort?

_____

_____

_____

Suggested Target Behaviors:

- I tend to only acknowledge success when there's a big outcome.
- I'm hard on myself for small mistakes.
- I often forget to recognize the effort I put in.
- I don't always notice the small steps that show real progress.
- I hold myself to unrealistic standards and call it "motivation."

My Target Behavior for Today

_____

⬛ Suggested Activity (3 Steps)

- Choose one thing you attempted today, even if it didn't go perfectly.
- Write down the effort it required—be honest and specific.
- Say or write a statement of pride: "I'm proud that I ___."

■ Evaluation System
Did I celebrate effort, not just outcome?

● Green (Named Effort + Felt Proud): I acknowledged what I did.
● Yellow (Wrote It, Didn't Feel It): I tried but felt unsure.
● Red (Ignored It): I didn't honor my effort today.

Reflection:

How can I keep noticing progress, even when it feels small or incomplete? Am I allowing space for growth, or am I getting stuck in rigid expectations? What does it look like to honor the process, not just the outcome, in line with my values?

_____

_____

_____

_____

_____

_____

Day 30

The Purpose Identity

🗨 Focus Skill: Identity Shaping

"Every action you take is a vote for the type of person you want to become"
- Thomas Jefferson

👤■ Target Behavior Identification

Where do I resist believing in my growth?

_____

_____

_____

Suggested Target Behaviors:

- I have been saying "I'm just not disciplined."
- I focus on flaws, not change.
- I don't notice my new habits.
- I downplay the small wins that show I'm growing.
- I define myself by old patterns instead of current effort.

My Target Behavior for Today

_____

■ Suggested Activity (3 Steps)

- Write a few "votes" you've cast for a disciplined identity this month (small habits, changes, moments).
- Create an identity statement: "I am someone who ___."
- Choose one way to reinforce that identity today.

■ Evaluation System

Did I connect my actions to my identity?

- ● Green (Named Identity + Reinforced It): I affirmed and acted as "that person."
- ● Yellow (Reflected, No Action): I thought about it but didn't follow through.
- ● Red (Didn't Reflect): I skipped this step.

Reflection:

Today, how did my actions reflect the kind of person I want to become? In what small ways did I move closer to what truly matters to me? What values showed up in my choices today — and where might I want to gently realign tomorrow?

_____

_____

_____

_____

_____

Executive Skills Development Questionnaire

This questionnaire assesses the development of executive skills like planning, decision-making, impulse control, and goal-directed behavior—key for managing tasks, emotions, and long-term success. Answer based on your experience; there are no right or wrong answers.

Note: This is not a diagnostic tool, but a guide to help identify areas to focus on in this journal.

Instructions:

For each statement, rate how frequently you experience the behavior or feeling described on a scale from 1 to 5:

1 = Never
2 = Rarely
3 = Sometimes
4 = Often
5 = Always

After completing the entire questionnaire, calculate the total score for each skill area and an overall executive functioning score. Higher scores indicate better development of that skill area.

I. Planning and Organization

Planning and organization skills help you manage time effectively, set goals, and break tasks into manageable steps. They are important for staying on track and meeting deadlines.

1. I create detailed plans for completing tasks and follow them.
2. I consistently set clear, achievable goals for myself
3. I use tools like planners, calendars, or digital reminders to stay organized.
4. I prioritize tasks based on urgency and importance.
5. I can break down large projects into smaller, manageable steps.
6. I stay organized and can manage multiple tasks simultaneously.
7. I create and organize spaces that enhance my focus and productivity.
8. I regularly track my progress toward goals and deadlines.

Planning and Organization Subtotal:
Total: (sum of scores for items 1-8)

II. Self-Regulation and Impulse Control

Self-regulation and impulse control involve the ability to manage your emotions, resist distractions, and make thoughtful decisions. This skill helps you stay focused on long-term goals and avoid reacting impulsively.

1. I stay calm in stressful situations and avoid reacting impulsively.
2. I resist temptations and stay focused on long-term goals.
3. I think before I react in emotionally charged situations.
4. I am able to delay immediate gratification to achieve a greater goal.
5. I handle frustration without it affecting my behavior.
6. I take a moment to pause and reflect before making important decisions.
7. I stay focused on tasks even when I am feeling distracted or anxious.
8. I am able to maintain self-control when faced with challenging emotions.

Self-Regulation and Impulse Control Subtotal:
Total: (sum of scores for items 1-8)

III. Working Memory

Working memory allows you to hold and manipulate information in your mind over short periods, which is essential for complex decision-making, multitasking, and problem-solving.

1. I can remember instructions or directions without needing to check them again.
2. I can keep track of multiple pieces of information at once.
3. I can recall details from past conversations or experiences when needed.
4. I use strategies to help me remember important information (e.g., repeating it to myself).
5. I can remember the main points of meetings or discussions without taking notes.
6. I can handle several tasks at once without forgetting key details.
7. I can retain information for long enough to solve a problem or complete a task.
8. I recall necessary information quickly when I need it.

Working Memory Subtotal:
Total: (sum of scores for items 1-8)

IV. Cognitive Flexibility

Cognitive flexibility is the ability to adapt your thinking and behavior when confronted with new information, challenges, or changes. It allows you to switch between tasks or perspectives with ease.

1. I can easily switch between tasks without losing focus.
2. I am comfortable adjusting my plans or strategies when unexpected events arise.
3. I am able to consider multiple perspectives when solving a problem.
4. I can let go of unhelpful thoughts or strategies and try new approaches.
5. I find it easy to adapt to changes in routine or plans.
6. I can change my thinking quickly when I encounter new information.
7. I approach problems with an open mind and am willing to experiment with different solutions.
8. I don't get stuck on one way of thinking and can shift my approach when needed.

Cognitive Flexibility Subtotal:
Total: (sum of scores for items 1-8)

V. Emotional Regulation

Emotional regulation involves the ability to understand and manage your emotions in a healthy way, especially during stress or conflict. It helps you remain composed and make thoughtful decisions.

1. I can identify and name my emotions as they arise.
2. I am able to stay calm and composed in stressful or frustrating situations.
3. I can manage my emotions without letting them affect my behavior.
4. I use coping strategies (e.g., deep breathing, mindfulness) to calm myself down.
5. I can remain focused on my tasks even when I'm feeling anxious or upset.
6. I communicate my emotions clearly to others without becoming defensive or overly emotional.
7. I recover quickly from setbacks and don't let negative emotions interfere with my progress.
8. I recognize when I'm overwhelmed and take steps to self-soothe.

Emotional Regulation Subtotal:
Total: (sum of scores for items 1-8)

VI. Decision-Making and Problem-Solving

Decision-making and problem-solving involve evaluating options, weighing pros and cons, and choosing the best course of action. These skills also help you come up with creative solutions when faced with challenges.

1. I weigh multiple options before making decisions.
2. I consider both short-term and long-term consequences when making decisions.
3. I feel confident in my ability to solve problems, even when they are complex.
4. I break problems into smaller, more manageable parts to find solutions.
5. I seek feedback from others when making important decisions.
6. I use critical thinking to evaluate the information available to me.
7. I trust my judgment when making decisions, even under pressure.
8. I approach challenges with a problem-solving mindset, focusing on finding solutions.

Decision-Making and Problem-Solving Subtotal:
Total: (sum of scores for items 1-8)

VII. Goal Setting and Achievement

Goal setting and achievement involve identifying meaningful objectives, breaking them into actionable steps, and working toward them persistently. This skill helps you stay motivated and track your progress.

- I set clear, measurable goals for myself in both personal and professional contexts.
- I break larger goals into smaller, more achievable steps.
- I regularly review my goals to ensure I'm staying on track.
- I remain focused on my goals, even when faced with challenges.
- I celebrate small milestones along the way to reaching my goals.
- I persist and continue working toward my goals, even when progress is slow.
- I adjust my goals when necessary to keep them realistic and achievable.
- I use setbacks as learning experiences and don't let them derail my progress.

Goal Setting and Achievement Subtotal:
Total: (sum of scores for items 1-8)

VIII. Attention and Focus

Attention and focus are essential for maintaining concentration on tasks over time, especially when there are distractions. This skill helps you stay productive and complete tasks efficiently.

- I can maintain focus on a task for long periods without becoming distracted.
- I use strategies (e.g., time blocking, minimizing distractions) to stay focused.
- I avoid multitasking and focus on one task at a time.
- I can maintain my attention on complex tasks without losing track.
- I notice when my attention starts to drift and refocus myself quickly.
- I consistently complete tasks in a timely manner.
- I can block out external distractions (e.g., noise, interruptions) when working on important tasks.
- I feel confident in my ability to stay on task until I complete it.

Attention and Focus Subtotal:
Total: (sum of scores for items 1-8)

Interpretation of Subskill Scores

Each skill area has a different range based on the responses to its individual items. Here's how to interpret the subskill scores:

1. Planning and Organization:
- 8-16 (Emerging): Difficulty with setting and organizing goals; may need structure and tools to improve.
- 17-24 (Developing): Basic organizational skills are present, but additional practice in planning and prioritizing may be beneficial.
- 25-32 (Proficient): Strong skills in organizing tasks, setting goals, and managing time effectively.
- 33-40 (Advanced): Highly developed organizational skills; able to manage complex tasks and prioritize effectively.
-

2. Self-Regulation and Impulse Control:
- 8-16 (Emerging): May struggle with emotional control and impulse regulation in stressful situations.
- 17-24 (Developing): Shows some capacity to regulate impulses and emotions, but more practice is needed under pressure.
- 25-32 (Proficient): Able to stay calm and think before reacting, even in challenging situations.
- 33-40 (Advanced): Excellent self-regulation; remains composed, manages stress well, and is able to delay gratification consistently.

3. Working Memory:
- 8-16 (Emerging): Difficulty holding and recalling information; may need strategies to improve memory.
- 17-24 (Developing): Can retain some information but may forget details under pressure.
- 25-32 (Proficient): Able to recall and manage information effectively, even when multitasking.
- 33-40 (Advanced): Excellent memory retention; able to handle complex information and recall details with ease.

4. Cognitive Flexibility:

- 8-16 (Emerging): Struggles with adapting to changes; tends to fixate on one approach.
- 17-24 (Developing): Can adapt to changes but may find it difficult in unfamiliar or stressful situations.
- 25-32 (Proficient): Able to switch between tasks and perspectives effectively.
- 33-40 (Advanced): Highly flexible; can change approaches with ease and handle unexpected situations confidently.

5. Emotional Regulation:

- 8-16 (Emerging): Difficulty managing emotions; prone to emotional outbursts or frustration.
- 17-24 (Developing): Can regulate emotions in some situations but struggles in highly stressful ones.
- 25-32 (Proficient): Manages emotions well and remains calm during challenges.
- 33-40 (Advanced): Strong emotional regulation; remains balanced, even in emotionally charged situations

6. Decision-Making and Problem-Solving:

- 8-16 (Emerging): Difficulty making decisions; may avoid problem-solving or feel overwhelmed by options.
- 17-24 (Developing): Can make basic decisions but may struggle with more complex or high-stakes choices.
- 25-32 (Proficient): Confident in making decisions and solving problems effectively.
- 33-40 (Advanced): Highly effective decision-making and problem-solving skills; able to analyze complex situations and choose the best course of action.

7. Goal Setting and Achievement:

- 8-16 (Emerging): Struggles with setting clear goals or following through with plans.
- 17-24 (Developing): Sets goals but may struggle with consistency or tracking progress.
- 25-32 (Proficient): Strong goal-setting skills; regularly tracks progress and makes adjustments as needed.
- 33-40 (Advanced): Highly effective goal setter; consistently achieves goals and adapts to changing circumstances.

8. Attention and Focus:

- 8-16 (Emerging): Frequently distracted; struggles with maintaining focus for extended periods.
- 17-24 (Developing): Can maintain focus but may get distracted in certain environments or tasks.
- 25-32 (Proficient): Able to focus on tasks for extended periods and manage distractions well.
- 33-40 (Advanced): Excellent attention and focus; remains fully engaged with tasks even in high-distraction environments.

Congratulations!

You've completed your 30-day journey to self-empowerment— built on small wins and self-compassion.
This wasn't about perfection but about showing up, noticing your habits, and making choices aligned with who you're becoming.

⅄ What now?

- Revisit the journal. Keep using your favorite prompts or mix them up as needed.
- Make it personal. Create your own prompts, like:
  - "What's one thing I'm proud of today?"
  - "Where did I show up for myself?"
- Use what worked. Stick with the tools or habits that helped you most.
- Watch for old patterns. All-or-nothing thinking may pop up, but that's normal. Respond with patience.
- Find your rhythm. You don't need daily journaling — weekly check-ins or voice notes might work better for you.

💬 Final Reflection:

You've shown up for yourself over these 30 days — not to be perfect, but to be present. Through each reflection and practice, you've gently shifted your habits, mindset, and responses in ways that align with your values and who you're becoming. Self-discipline isn't about control or rigidity — it's about returning, again and again, to what truly matters. It's about creating an environment that supports your goals and makes it easier to live in alignment, even when life feels messy.
Progress isn't linear. Some days will feel easier than others, and that's not failure — it's feedback. Let those moments be invitations to pause, reflect, and adjust with grace. This journal is not a checklist but a companion — something you can return to whenever you need to reconnect, reset, or renew your intentions. You're not starting over; you're continuing forward, equipped with more awareness, self-compassion, and clarity than before.

🚀 Keep going. Keep returning. Keep becoming. ✸